CONTENTS

INTRODUCTION

In a world where culinary delights have the power to transcend boundaries and bring people together, there exists a unique and often overlooked challenge: dysphagia. This condition, affecting millions worldwide, hampers the joy of eating by impairing the ability to swallow. However, within this adversity lies an opportunity for innovation, creativity, and the transformation of mealtimes into extraordinary experiences. Welcome to "Taste and Triumph: Exploring the Ultramodern Dysphagia Cookbook."

In this groundbreaking culinary journey, we embark on a quest to redefine the boundaries of flavor, texture, and presentation, empowering individuals with dysphagia to savor the pleasures of food once again. Gone are the days of dull, pureed meals and monotonous dietary restrictions. Instead, we delve into a world where cutting-edge techniques, pioneering ingredients, and artistic plating techniques converge to create a symphony of taste and visual delight.

"Ultramodern Dysphagia Cookbook" is not just another cookbook. It is a testament to the resilience and ingenuity of individuals facing the daily challenges of dysphagia. It is a tribute to their unwavering spirit, proving that no obstacle is insurmountable when passion and creativity collide. By blending the art of gastronomy with scientific understanding, this book aims to revolutionize the way we approach dysphagia management, enabling individuals to nourish both body and soul.

Within these pages, you will discover a treasure trove

of recipes meticulously crafted to meet the unique needs of those with dysphagia. Each dish combines innovative thickening agents, advanced cooking techniques, and thoughtfully curated ingredients to transform ordinary ingredients into extraordinary culinary masterpieces. From velvety soups and succulent main courses to tantalizing desserts and delightful beverages, the recipes presented here encompass a world of flavors that will captivate the senses and awaken a renewed love for food.

But this cookbook is more than just a collection of recipes. It is a comprehensive guide that educates, empowers, and embraces the dysphagia community. You will find practical tips, expert advice, and a wealth of knowledge about dysphagia management, including the latest research and developments in the field. With an unwavering commitment to inclusivity, we strive to make this cookbook a valuable resource for caregivers, healthcare professionals, and anyone seeking to support individuals on their journey to regain culinary joy.

So, join us as we embark on this extraordinary gastronomic adventure, celebrating the triumph of taste over adversity. Together, let us rewrite the narrative of dysphagia, fostering a world where everyone can savor the magic of food, regardless of the challenges they face. Get ready to immerse yourself in the wonders of "Taste and Triumph: Exploring the Ultramodern Dysphagia Cookbook."

CHAPTER ONE

Introduction
a. What is dysphagia?

Dysphagia is a medical condition characterized by difficulty or discomfort in swallowing. It can affect people of all ages, from infants to the elderly, and can be caused by various factors, including neurological disorders, muscular disorders, structural abnormalities, or even as a side effect of certain medications. Dysphagia can have a significant impact on an individual's ability to eat and drink, leading to a range of physical and emotional challenges.

There are two main types of dysphagia: oropharyngeal dysphagia and esophageal dysphagia. Oropharyngeal dysphagia occurs when there is a problem with the muscles and nerves involved in swallowing, often resulting in difficulty in moving food from the mouth to the throat. Esophageal dysphagia, on the other hand, occurs when there are issues with the esophagus, such as narrowing or blockage, making it challenging for food to pass through to the stomach.

Dysphagia can cause a variety of symptoms, including choking, coughing or gagging during meals, a sensation of food getting stuck in the throat or chest, regurgitation, weight loss, and even respiratory problems. These symptoms can significantly impact an individual's quality of life, leading to social isolation, malnutrition, dehydration, and a decline in overall health.

b. Importance of nutrition for individuals with dysphagia

Nutrition plays a crucial role in the overall health and

well-being of individuals with dysphagia. Since swallowing difficulties can lead to reduced intake of food and fluids, it is important to ensure that individuals with dysphagia receive adequate nutrition to meet their dietary needs. Proper nutrition can help maintain strength, prevent malnutrition, improve energy levels, and support overall health.

Individuals with dysphagia often require modified diets, which may involve altering the texture, consistency, or viscosity of food and fluids. These modifications are aimed at making swallowing safer and more manageable. Some common modifications include pureeing foods, thickening liquids, or choosing foods that naturally have a softer texture. It is important to work closely with a healthcare professional, such as a speech-language pathologist or dietitian, to determine the appropriate modifications for each individual's specific needs.

In addition to modifications, nutritional supplements can also be beneficial for individuals with dysphagia. These supplements can provide additional calories, protein, vitamins, and minerals to help meet nutritional requirements. They are available in various forms, such as powders, liquids, or bars, and can be tailored to an individual's specific dietary needs.

c. Challenges faced by individuals with dysphagia in meal preparation

Meal preparation can become a significant challenge for individuals with dysphagia. The need for modified textures and consistencies, as well as the potential for certain foods to trigger swallowing difficulties, can make it difficult to plan and prepare meals that are both safe and enjoyable.

Here are some challenges commonly faced by individuals with dysphagia in meal preparation:

- Texture modifications: Modifying the texture of food to meet specific swallowing requirements can be time-consuming and may require specialized kitchen equipment, such as blenders or food processors. It can be challenging to achieve the desired texture while still preserving the taste and nutritional value of the food.
- Limited food choices: Some foods may pose a higher risk of choking or discomfort for individuals with dysphagia. This limitation in food choices can make meal planning more challenging and may lead to a monotonous or repetitive diet.
- Finding dysphagia-friendly recipes: It can be challenging to find recipes that are specifically designed for individuals with dysphagia. Many traditional recipes may need to be modified or adapted, and it may require creativity and experimentation to develop flavorful and appealing meals.
- Emotional impact: Mealtime is often associated with socializing, pleasure, and enjoyment. However, individuals with dysphagia may experience anxiety or frustration around meals due to the challenges they face. It is important to address the emotional impact of dysphagia and provide support to help individuals maintain a positive relationship with food.

d. How this cookbook can help improve their quality of life

A specialized cookbook designed for individuals with dysphagia can be a valuable resource in improving their quality of life. Such a cookbook can provide a wide range of dysphagia-friendly recipes, tips, and guidance to help individuals with dysphagia and their caregivers in meal preparation.

Here are some ways in which a dysphagia cookbook can be beneficial:

- Variety of recipes: The cookbook can offer a diverse selection of recipes that are modified to meet the needs of individuals with dysphagia. These recipes can cover different meal types, including breakfast, lunch, dinner, and snacks, ensuring a broader range of choices and reducing the monotony of the diet.
- Clear instructions: The cookbook can provide detailed instructions on how to modify the textures of various foods and create dysphagia-friendly meals. This can help individuals and caregivers understand the process and make the necessary modifications with confidence.
- Nutritional information: A dysphagia cookbook can provide nutritional information for each recipe, including calorie and nutrient content. This information is crucial for individuals with dysphagia to ensure they are meeting their dietary needs and maintaining proper nutrition.
- Tips and techniques: The cookbook can offer helpful tips and techniques for meal preparation, such as alternative ingredients, cooking methods, and presentation ideas. These tips can enhance the overall dining experience and make meals

more enjoyable.

- Support and inspiration: By providing a collection of dysphagia-friendly recipes, the cookbook can offer support and inspiration to individuals with dysphagia and their caregivers. It can help them explore new flavors, rediscover familiar dishes, and foster a positive attitude towards mealtime.

In conclusion, dysphagia is a medical condition characterized by difficulty in swallowing, which can have significant impacts on an individual's ability to eat and drink. Nutrition plays a vital role in supporting the health and well-being of individuals with dysphagia. However, meal preparation can present numerous challenges, including texture modifications, limited food choices, and emotional impact. A specialized dysphagia cookbook can help address these challenges by providing a variety of dysphagia-friendly recipes, clear instructions, nutritional information, helpful tips, and support. By using this cookbook as a resource, individuals with dysphagia can improve their quality of life and enjoy safe and satisfying meals.

Understanding Dysphagia
a. Different types and causes of dysphagia

Dysphagia can be classified into two main types: oropharyngeal dysphagia and esophageal dysphagia. Each type has different causes and affects different parts of the swallowing process.

Oropharyngeal dysphagia: This type of dysphagia occurs when there is a problem with the muscles and nerves involved in swallowing, mainly in the mouth and throat. It can be caused by various factors, including:

- Neurological disorders: Conditions such as stroke, Parkinson's disease, multiple sclerosis, or amyotrophic lateral sclerosis (ALS) can affect the nerves and muscles responsible for swallowing.
- Structural abnormalities: Structural issues in the oral or pharyngeal area, such as tumors, cleft palate, or damage to the head or neck, can lead to oropharyngeal dysphagia.
- Muscle disorders: Certain muscular conditions, like muscular dystrophy or myasthenia gravis, can weaken the muscles involved in swallowing.
- Aging: As people age, the muscles used for swallowing may weaken, leading to oropharyngeal dysphagia.

Esophageal dysphagia: This type of dysphagia occurs when there are problems with the esophagus, the tube that carries food from the throat to the stomach. Some common causes of esophageal dysphagia include:

- Gastroesophageal reflux disease (GERD): Chronic acid reflux can lead to inflammation and narrowing of the esophagus, causing difficulty in swallowing.
- Esophageal strictures: Narrowing of the esophagus due to scar tissue formation can result from conditions like gastroesophageal reflux disease, long-term use of a feeding tube, or radiation therapy.
- Achalasia: This condition occurs when the lower esophageal sphincter (the muscular ring that allows food to enter the stomach) doesn't relax properly, making it difficult for food to pass through.

- Tumors or cancer: Benign or malignant growths in the esophagus can obstruct the passage of food.
- Esophageal motility disorders: Conditions that affect the normal contractions and movements of the esophagus, such as diffuse esophageal spasm or scleroderma, can lead to esophageal dysphagia.

b. The swallowing process and its complications

Swallowing, also known as deglutition, is a complex process that involves coordination between various muscles and nerves. It can be divided into three main phases: the oral phase, pharyngeal phase, and esophageal phase. Complications can arise at any stage of the swallowing process, leading to dysphagia.

Oral phase: The oral phase begins with the preparation of food in the mouth and ends when the tongue pushes the food to the back of the throat. Complications during this phase can include:

- Poor tongue control or weakness: Weak or uncoordinated tongue movements can make it difficult to propel the food backward.
- Chewing difficulties: Problems with biting, chewing, or manipulating food can hinder the formation of a cohesive bolus for swallowing.
- Reduced saliva production: Insufficient saliva can make it harder to form a moist bolus that can be swallowed easily.

Pharyngeal phase: The pharyngeal phase starts when the bolus of food enters the throat and ends when it reaches the esophagus. Complications during this phase can include:

- Weak or uncoordinated throat muscles:

Inadequate muscle strength or coordination can result in food getting stuck in the throat or entering the airway.

- Impaired swallowing reflex: If the swallowing reflex is delayed or absent, food may enter the airway instead of the esophagus.
- Dysfunctional upper esophageal sphincter: The upper esophageal sphincter, which opens to allow food into the esophagus, may not function properly, leading to difficulty in food passage.

Esophageal phase: The esophageal phase begins as the food enters the esophagus and ends when it reaches the stomach. Complications during this phase can include:

- Esophageal narrowing or obstruction: Narrowing of the esophagus due to strictures, tumors, or other abnormalities can hinder the smooth passage of food.
- Weakened esophageal contractions: Inadequate contractions of the esophageal muscles can cause food to move slowly through the esophagus or get stuck.
- Gastroesophageal reflux: Acid reflux can irritate the esophagus, causing inflammation and making swallowing uncomfortable.

c. Common symptoms and challenges associated with dysphagia

Dysphagia can present a range of symptoms and challenges that can significantly impact an individual's daily life and overall well-being.

- Difficulty in swallowing: The most apparent symptom of dysphagia is difficulty in swallowing.

It may feel as if food or liquids are getting stuck in the throat or chest.

- Choking or coughing: Individuals with dysphagia may experience episodes of choking or coughing while eating or drinking, especially if the food or liquid enters the airway.
- Regurgitation: Some individuals may experience regurgitation, where swallowed food comes back up into the mouth or throat.
- Weight loss and malnutrition: Dysphagia can lead to reduced food intake, resulting in weight loss and nutritional deficiencies. This can further impact overall health and energy levels.
- Dehydration: Difficulties in drinking liquids can lead to inadequate fluid intake, causing dehydration.
- Respiratory problems: If food or liquids enter the airway, it can lead to respiratory issues, such as aspiration pneumonia or recurrent chest infections.
- Social and emotional challenges: Dysphagia can affect an individual's social interactions and emotional well-being. It may lead to anxiety or embarrassment related to eating in public, and individuals may feel isolated or limited in their ability to enjoy meals with friends and family.
- Increased mealtime duration: The need for careful chewing, swallowing techniques, and modified textures can significantly prolong mealtime, making it more time-consuming.
- Impact on quality of life: The challenges associated with dysphagia can impact an individual's overall quality of life, including their

ability to enjoy food, participate in social events, and maintain a sense of independence.

Understanding the types, causes, swallowing process, and challenges associated with dysphagia is crucial in providing appropriate support and management for individuals living with this condition. Collaborating with healthcare professionals, such as speech-language pathologists, dietitians, and physicians, can help develop personalized strategies to address these challenges and improve the well-being of individuals with dysphagia.

Dietary Guidelines for Dysphagia

a. Texture modification techniques for safe swallowing

Texture modification is an essential aspect of managing dysphagia and ensuring safe swallowing. Modifying the texture of food and liquids can help individuals with dysphagia consume meals more easily. Here are some common texture modification techniques:

- Pureed: Foods are blended until they reach a smooth, pudding-like consistency. This texture is suitable for individuals with severe swallowing difficulties who require minimal effort to swallow.
- Minced and moist: Foods are finely chopped into small, soft, and moist pieces. This texture helps individuals with moderate swallowing difficulties who can manage some texture but still require minimal effort to swallow.
- Soft and bite-sized: Foods are cooked until tender and cut into bite-sized pieces. This texture is suitable for individuals with mild swallowing difficulties who can handle slightly more texture but still need to avoid hard or crunchy foods.

- Thickened liquids: Liquids are thickened using thickeners, such as commercial thickeners or natural thickeners like gelatin or starch. Thickened liquids are easier to control in the mouth and reduce the risk of aspiration.

It's important to note that texture modifications should be tailored to individual needs. Working with a speech-language pathologist or dietitian is crucial to determine the appropriate texture modification techniques and ensure nutritional needs are met.

b. Nutritional requirements for individuals with dysphagia

Meeting nutritional requirements is crucial for individuals with dysphagia to maintain overall health and prevent malnutrition. Here are some key considerations for their nutritional needs:

- Adequate calorie intake: Dysphagia can lead to reduced food intake, so it's important to ensure individuals with dysphagia consume enough calories to meet their energy requirements. This may involve choosing high-calorie options or adding nutritional supplements.
- Protein: Protein is essential for tissue repair and maintenance. Including protein-rich foods, such as lean meats, fish, poultry, legumes, and dairy products, is important to meet protein needs.
- Vitamins and minerals: A varied and balanced diet is necessary to ensure individuals with dysphagia receive essential vitamins and minerals. Including a wide range of fruits, vegetables, whole grains, and dairy or dairy alternatives can help meet

these requirements.

- Fiber: Adequate fiber intake is important for digestive health. While texture modifications may limit fiber intake, including pureed or soft fruits and vegetables, as well as incorporating fiber supplements if needed, can help maintain bowel regularity.
- Hydration: Maintaining proper hydration is crucial for individuals with dysphagia. If thin liquids pose a swallowing challenge, using thickened liquids or consuming foods with high water content, such as soups or fruits, can help meet hydration needs.

It is important to consult with a dietitian who specializes in dysphagia management to develop an individualized meal plan that meets the specific nutritional needs of individuals with dysphagia.

c. Food and liquid consistencies suitable for different levels of dysphagia

Different levels of dysphagia require specific food and liquid consistencies to ensure safe swallowing. The International Dysphagia Diet Standardisation Initiative (IDDSI) framework provides a standardized system for categorizing food and liquid consistencies. Here are the consistencies suitable for different levels of dysphagia:

- Level 0 - Thin liquids: This includes unthickened water, juice, milk, and other fluids that are thin in consistency. Individuals with mild dysphagia or no swallowing difficulties can typically tolerate thin liquids without modifications.
- Level 1 - Slightly thick liquids: Liquids at

this level have a slightly thicker consistency to minimize the risk of aspiration. They should flow slowly off a spoon and require minimal effort to swallow. These can be achieved using commercial thickeners or natural thickeners like gelatin or starch.

- Level 2 - Mildly thick liquids: Liquids at this level are thicker than Level 1, resembling the consistency of nectar. They pour off a spoon in a controlled manner and require slightly more effort to swallow.
- Level 3 - Moderately thick liquids: These liquids have a consistency similar to honey. They flow off a spoon more slowly and require more effort to swallow.
- Level 4 - Pureed: Foods at this level have a smooth, cohesive, pudding-like consistency. They should maintain their shape on a spoon but can be easily mashed with gentle pressure.
- Level 5 - Minced and moist: Foods at this level are finely chopped into small, soft, and moist pieces. They should be manageable with minimal chewing and effort.
- Level 6 - Soft and bite-sized: Foods at this level are cooked until tender and cut into bite-sized pieces. They should be soft enough to be easily chewed and require minimal effort to swallow.

It's important to note that the appropriate food and liquid consistencies should be determined through a swallowing evaluation conducted by a speech-language pathologist, who can assess an individual's swallowing abilities and recommend the appropriate consistency level.

d. Safety precautions and considerations while preparing dysphagia-friendly meals

When preparing dysphagia-friendly meals, it is important to follow specific safety precautions and considerations to ensure the food is safe to swallow. Here are some key guidelines to keep in mind:

- Modify food textures: Use appropriate texture modification techniques, such as pureeing, mincing, or softening foods, based on the individual's swallowing abilities and recommendations from healthcare professionals.
- Avoid dry and crumbly foods: Dry and crumbly foods, such as crackers or chips, can be difficult to swallow. Choose moist and cohesive foods that are easier to form into boluses and swallow safely.
- Eliminate hard or tough-to-chew foods: Foods that require excessive chewing or have tough textures, like raw vegetables or tough meats, should be avoided. Opt for softer alternatives that are easier to chew and swallow.
- Ensure proper food consistency: Consistencies should be uniform throughout the meal to avoid confusion and potential choking hazards. Ensure that all food items, including side dishes and sauces, have the appropriate texture modification.
- Consider flavor and nutrition: While focusing on texture modification, aim to preserve flavor and nutritional value. Use herbs, spices, and seasonings to enhance the taste of dysphagia-friendly meals without compromising safety.
- Serve at an appropriate temperature: Extreme temperatures can be discomforting and increase

the risk of aspiration. Serve meals at a safe temperature that is comfortable for the individual.

- Maintain hygiene and food safety: Follow proper food handling and hygiene practices to reduce the risk of foodborne illnesses. This includes washing hands thoroughly, sanitizing cooking utensils and surfaces, and storing food at safe temperatures.

- Consider individual preferences: Take into account the individual's personal preferences and dietary restrictions when preparing dysphagia-friendly meals. This can help improve the overall satisfaction and enjoyment of the dining experience.

By adhering to these safety precautions and considerations, caregivers and individuals with dysphagia can ensure that meals are prepared in a manner that promotes safe swallowing and optimal nutrition while still catering to personal tastes and preferences.

Modified Diets and Special Considerations

a. Specific dietary modifications for different medical conditions

Dietary modifications play a crucial role in managing various medical conditions. Here are some specific dietary modifications for common medical conditions:

- Diabetes: For individuals with diabetes, it is important to monitor carbohydrate intake to manage blood sugar levels. This may involve portion control, choosing complex carbohydrates with a lower glycemic index, and balancing meals with a combination of carbohydrates, protein, and healthy fats.

- Hypertension (High Blood Pressure): A low-sodium diet is often recommended for individuals with hypertension. This involves reducing salt intake by avoiding processed foods, using herbs and spices to season meals instead of salt, and choosing fresh ingredients.
- Celiac Disease: Individuals with celiac disease need to follow a gluten-free diet. This means avoiding foods containing wheat, barley, rye, and their derivatives. Gluten-free alternatives, such as rice, quinoa, and gluten-free flours, can be used in recipes.
- Food Allergies: Dietary modifications are necessary for individuals with food allergies. This involves avoiding specific allergens, such as peanuts, tree nuts, shellfish, dairy, or eggs. Reading food labels carefully and substituting allergenic ingredients with suitable alternatives is important.
- Gastroesophageal Reflux Disease (GERD): Individuals with GERD often benefit from a low-acid diet. This includes avoiding acidic foods and beverages, such as citrus fruits, tomatoes, coffee, and carbonated drinks. It also involves consuming smaller, more frequent meals and avoiding lying down immediately after eating.
- Renal (Kidney) Disease: For individuals with renal disease, a renal diet is recommended to manage electrolyte levels and minimize stress on the kidneys. This may involve controlling protein, sodium, and potassium intake, and monitoring fluid consumption.

It is important to consult with healthcare professionals, such as registered dietitians or physicians, to develop an individualized dietary plan tailored to specific medical conditions.

b. Meal plans and recipes for common dietary restrictions (e.g., gluten-free, low-sodium)

When following specific dietary restrictions, meal planning and having access to suitable recipes is essential. Here are some tips for creating meal plans and finding recipes for common dietary restrictions:

- Gluten-Free: Look for gluten-free recipes that use naturally gluten-free ingredients like rice, quinoa, corn, and certified gluten-free oats. Opt for whole foods and explore gluten-free alternatives like gluten-free flours, bread, and pasta. Incorporate a variety of fruits, vegetables, lean proteins, and healthy fats.
- Low-Sodium: Create meal plans that focus on whole, unprocessed foods and limit the use of high-sodium ingredients. Use herbs, spices, and salt-free seasonings to add flavor to dishes. Choose fresh fruits and vegetables, lean proteins, whole grains, and low-sodium or no-added-salt products.
- Dairy-Free: Plan meals that avoid dairy products and use suitable alternatives like almond milk, coconut milk, or soy milk. Look for dairy-free recipes that use non-dairy sources of calcium and other nutrients, such as leafy greens, fortified plant-based products, and nuts.
- Vegetarian or Vegan: Incorporate a variety of

plant-based protein sources such as legumes, tofu, tempeh, quinoa, and nuts. Plan meals that are rich in fruits, vegetables, whole grains, and healthy fats. Explore vegetarian or vegan recipes that provide a balance of nutrients and flavors.

- Nut-Free: When creating meal plans for individuals with nut allergies, ensure that all recipes and ingredients are free from nuts and nut products. Be cautious of cross-contamination and read food labels carefully. Look for nut-free alternatives and substitutes to recreate favorite dishes.

To find meal plans and recipes for specific dietary restrictions, consider utilizing online resources, cookbooks dedicated to specific dietary needs, and consulting with registered dietitians who specialize in those areas. These resources can provide inspiration and guidance for creating delicious and nutritionally balanced meals that adhere to specific dietary restrictions.

c. Tips for adapting the cookbook's recipes to meet individual dietary needs

Adapting recipes to meet individual dietary needs is an important skill for individuals with specific dietary restrictions. Here are some tips for adapting recipes from the cookbook to accommodate different dietary needs:

- Identify key allergens or restricted ingredients: Review the recipe and identify any allergens or ingredients that need to be avoided. For example, if the recipe calls for wheat flour and the individual has celiac disease, a gluten-free flour blend can be used as a substitute.

- Explore suitable alternatives: Research and identify suitable alternatives for the restricted ingredients. For example, if a recipe includes dairy, explore non-dairy milk options like almond milk, coconut milk, or soy milk. Replace dairy-based cheeses with plant-based alternatives or nutritional yeast.
- Adjust seasonings and flavors: Modify seasonings and flavors to suit individual preferences and dietary restrictions. For example, reduce sodium content by using salt-free seasonings or herbs and spices to enhance flavor. Experiment with different herbs, spices, and condiments to add variety and depth to the dish.
- Modify cooking techniques: Adjust cooking techniques to reduce the use of unhealthy fats or oils. For example, instead of frying, consider baking, grilling, or steaming. This helps reduce overall calorie intake and promote healthier cooking methods.
- Portion control and nutritional balance: Consider portion sizes and nutritional balance while adapting recipes. Ensure that meals include a balance of macronutrients (carbohydrates, proteins, and fats) and are portioned appropriately for individual needs.
- Seek guidance from professionals: If unsure about specific adaptations or dietary requirements, consult with registered dietitians or healthcare professionals who specialize in the specific dietary needs. They can provide guidance and advice tailored to individual requirements.

By using these tips and adapting recipes accordingly,

individuals can enjoy the variety of dishes in the cookbook while adhering to their specific dietary needs. Experimenting with substitutions, flavors, and cooking techniques can create delicious meals that accommodate dietary restrictions without compromising on taste and nutrition.

Managing Dysphagia Challenges
a. Strategies for overcoming common obstacles in dysphagia meal preparation

Meal preparation can pose challenges for individuals with dysphagia, but with the right strategies, these obstacles can be overcome. Here are some strategies to help overcome common obstacles in dysphagia meal preparation:

- Plan ahead: Plan meals in advance to ensure you have the necessary ingredients and equipment on hand. Consider batch cooking or meal prepping to save time and effort.
- Use convenience foods: Opt for pre-cut fruits and vegetables, pre-cooked proteins, or frozen vegetables that can be easily incorporated into meals. This can reduce the time and effort required for meal preparation.
- Seek assistance: If possible, enlist the help of a caregiver or family member to assist with meal preparation. This can involve chopping ingredients, setting up equipment, or following recipes under supervision.
- Modify cooking techniques: Explore cooking techniques that make food easier to swallow. For example, steaming or poaching can result in softer and more tender textures. Use a blender or

food processor to puree or blend ingredients for smoother textures.

- Use adaptive utensils and tools: Consider using specialized utensils and tools designed for individuals with swallowing difficulties. These may include angled or weighted utensils, non-slip cutting boards, or adaptive food processors. These tools can make meal preparation easier and safer.
- Experiment with texture modifications: Try different texture modification techniques, such as pureeing, mincing, or softening foods, to find the most suitable options for safe swallowing. Work with a speech-language pathologist or dietitian to determine the appropriate modifications.
- Incorporate variety and flavor: Dysphagia-friendly meals can still be flavorful and diverse. Experiment with herbs, spices, and seasonings to enhance the taste of meals. Explore different recipes and cuisines to keep meals interesting and enjoyable.

b. Tips for involving family members and caregivers in the cooking process

Involving family members and caregivers in the cooking process can foster a sense of collaboration and support. Here are some tips for involving them in dysphagia meal preparation:

- Communication and education: Clearly communicate the challenges and specific dietary needs associated with dysphagia to family members and caregivers. Educate them about the texture modifications, dietary restrictions, and safety precautions required.

- Delegate tasks: Assign specific tasks to family members or caregivers based on their capabilities and availability. This can include ingredient preparation, setting up equipment, or assisting with measuring and mixing ingredients.
- Provide guidance and instructions: Offer clear instructions and guidance on how to modify recipes and adhere to specific dietary requirements. Provide written recipes or visual aids to help them follow the process accurately.
- Share resources and recipes: Share educational resources, cookbooks, or online sources that offer dysphagia-friendly recipes and meal ideas. Encourage family members and caregivers to explore and experiment with these resources.
- Foster a supportive environment: Create an environment that encourages open communication, patience, and understanding. Appreciate their efforts and provide positive reinforcement for their involvement in the cooking process.
- Offer training or demonstrations: If needed, provide training or demonstrations on specific techniques or adaptations required for dysphagia meal preparation. This can help family members and caregivers feel more confident and capable in assisting with meal preparation.

c. Advice on maintaining a positive mindset and finding joy in cooking despite challenges

Cooking can be a source of joy and creativity, even in the face of challenges posed by dysphagia. Here are some tips to maintain a positive mindset and find joy in cooking:

- Embrace experimentation: View dysphagia-friendly cooking as an opportunity to explore new ingredients, flavors, and cooking techniques. Embrace the challenge of creating delicious and visually appealing meals within the constraints of the dietary restrictions.
- Focus on what can be enjoyed: Instead of dwelling on the limitations, focus on the wide variety of foods that can still be enjoyed. Experiment with different combinations of flavors, textures, and seasonings to create unique and tasty dishes.
- Seek inspiration: Explore dysphagia-friendly recipes, cookbooks, and online resources for inspiration. Join online communities or support groups where individuals share their experiences, tips, and recipe ideas. Engage with others who face similar challenges and exchange ideas.
- Make it a social activity: Involve family members, friends, or caregivers in the cooking process. Cook together, share stories, and create memories in the kitchen. Enjoy the social aspect of cooking and the sense of togetherness it can bring.
- Practice self-care: Take breaks, manage stress, and prioritize self-care. Cooking can be physically and emotionally demanding, so ensure you have time for relaxation and rejuvenation.
- Celebrate small victories: Acknowledge and celebrate each accomplishment, no matter how small. Whether it's mastering a new cooking technique or successfully creating a dysphagia-friendly meal, recognize and appreciate your efforts.

d. Meal Planning

Meal planning is a valuable tool for individuals with dysphagia, as it allows for organized and efficient meal preparation. Here are some tips for effective meal planning:

- Set aside dedicated time: Allocate a specific time each week to plan meals. This can be done on a day that works best for you, considering factors such as grocery shopping schedules and personal commitments.
- Consider individual preferences and dietary needs: Take into account personal preferences, dietary restrictions, and nutritional requirements when planning meals. Ensure a balance of nutrients by incorporating a variety of food groups.
- Plan for texture modifications: Keep in mind the recommended texture modifications for safe swallowing. Choose recipes and ingredients that can be easily modified to the appropriate texture levels.
- Create a meal calendar or weekly menu: Use a calendar or template to map out meals for the week. Include breakfast, lunch, dinner, and snacks, as well as dysphagia-friendly modifications. This visual aid can help you stay organized and ensure variety in your meals.
- Prep ingredients in advance: To streamline the meal preparation process, consider prepping ingredients ahead of time. Wash, chop, and portion ingredients as needed, storing them appropriately for freshness.
- Batch cooking and freezing: Prepare larger

quantities of dysphagia-friendly meals and freeze individual portions. This can save time and effort on busy days when you may not have the energy to cook from scratch.

- Make a shopping list: Based on your meal plan, create a shopping list to ensure you have all the necessary ingredients on hand. Check your pantry and fridge for any items that need to be replenished.
- Stay flexible and adaptable: Be prepared to make adjustments to your meal plan based on changing circumstances or unexpected events. Have backup options or quick and easy meals for days when time is limited.

By incorporating meal planning into your routine, you can alleviate stress, ensure proper nutrition, and streamline the process of dysphagia-friendly meal preparation.

Here's a sample 7-day meal plan for individuals with dysphagia. Please note that this is a general meal plan, and it's important to customize it based on individual dietary restrictions, texture modifications, and specific nutritional needs.

Day 1:

- Breakfast: Scrambled eggs with pureed spinach and mashed avocado
- Lunch: Pureed chicken and vegetable soup
- Dinner: Baked salmon with mashed sweet potatoes and pureed green beans
- Snack: Pureed fruit smoothie

Day 2:

- Breakfast: Smoothie with yogurt, banana, and

pureed strawberries
- Lunch: Pureed lentil soup with soft-textured bread
- Dinner: Pureed beef stew with mashed carrots and peas
- Snack: Pureed mango with yogurt

Day 3:

- Breakfast: Oatmeal with pureed peaches and ground cinnamon
- Lunch: Pureed turkey and vegetable meatballs with soft-textured pasta
- Dinner: Pureed chicken curry with rice and pureed cauliflower
- Snack: Pureed pear with cottage cheese

Day 4:

- Breakfast: Pureed cottage cheese with mashed banana and cinnamon
- Lunch: Pureed broccoli and cheddar soup
- Dinner: Pureed meatloaf with mashed potatoes and pureed carrots
- Snack: Pureed blueberry yogurt

Day 5:

- Breakfast: Smoothie with yogurt, spinach, and pureed pineapple
- Lunch: Pureed black bean soup with soft-textured tortilla
- Dinner: Pureed salmon with mashed butternut squash and pureed asparagus
- Snack: Pureed watermelon with Greek yogurt

Day 6:

- Breakfast: Pureed scrambled eggs with mashed

avocado and pureed tomatoes
- Lunch: Pureed vegetable lasagna
- Dinner: Pureed turkey chili with mashed sweet potatoes
- Snack: Pureed peach with cottage cheese

Day 7:

- Breakfast: Oatmeal with pureed apples and ground cinnamon
- Lunch: Pureed chicken and rice soup
- Dinner: Pureed shrimp stir-fry with rice noodles and pureed zucchini
- Snack: Pureed strawberry yogurt

Remember to consult with a healthcare professional or registered dietitian to ensure that this meal plan aligns with individual dietary needs, texture modifications, and any specific medical conditions. They can provide personalized recommendations and further guidance for meal planning.

Conclusion

a. Recapecap of key takeaways and insights from the book

The cookbook for individuals with dysphagia offers valuable insights and key takeaways to enhance their meal experiences. Here is a recapecap of some key points from the book:

- Texture modifications: The book provides various techniques for modifying the texture of food to ensure safe swallowing. It emphasizes the importance of pureeing, mincing, or softening ingredients to create dysphagia-friendly meals.
- Nutritional considerations: The cookbook

highlights the significance of meeting nutritional requirements while managing dysphagia. It offers guidance on incorporating essential nutrients, vitamins, and minerals into modified meals to maintain overall health and well-being.

- Customization for dietary needs: The book acknowledges that individuals with dysphagia may have specific dietary restrictions or medical conditions. It provides tips on adapting recipes to meet various dietary needs, such as gluten-free, low-sodium, or diabetic-friendly options.
- Meal planning and organization: The cookbook emphasizes the importance of meal planning and organization to simplify the cooking process. It suggests creating meal calendars, prepping ingredients in advance, and utilizing batch cooking and freezing techniques.
- Involvement of caregivers and family members: The book recognizes the role of caregivers and family members in supporting individuals with dysphagia. It offers suggestions for involving them in the cooking process, fostering collaboration, and sharing the responsibility of meal preparation.
- Finding joy in cooking: Despite the challenges posed by dysphagia, the book encourages individuals to maintain a positive mindset and find joy in cooking. It promotes experimentation, flavor exploration, and the creation of visually appealing meals to enhance the overall dining experience.

b. Encouragement for individuals with dysphagia and

their caregivers

To individuals with dysphagia and their caregivers, I want to offer words of encouragement. Living with dysphagia can present daily challenges, but it's important to remember that you are not alone. Here are some words of encouragement:

- Stay positive: Remember that you have the strength and resilience to overcome challenges. Approach each day with a positive mindset, focusing on what you can achieve rather than dwelling on limitations.
- Seek support: Reach out to support groups, online communities, or local organizations that cater to individuals with dysphagia. Connect with others who face similar challenges and share experiences, tips, and encouragement.
- Celebrate small victories: Recognize and celebrate each achievement along your journey. Whether it's trying a new recipe, successfully modifying a meal, or finding joy in the cooking process, every step forward is worth celebrating.
- Practice self-care: Taking care of your physical, mental, and emotional well-being is crucial. Allow yourself moments of rest and relaxation, engage in activities you enjoy, and prioritize self-care to maintain balance and reduce stress.
- Communicate openly: Effective communication with healthcare professionals, speech-language pathologists, and dietitians is vital. Share your concerns, goals, and challenges with them to receive personalized guidance and support.
- Embrace teamwork: Engage your family

members, friends, and caregivers as a supportive team. Encourage their involvement in the cooking process, communicate your needs, and appreciate their efforts in assisting you.

Remember, every step you take toward improving your quality of life matters. You have the ability to adapt, find joy in the kitchen, and create delicious meals that meet your dietary needs.

c. Final thoughts on the importance of accessible and enjoyable meals for everyone

Accessible and enjoyable meals are essential for individuals with dysphagia and should be a priority for everyone. Here are some final thoughts on the importance of such meals:

- Nutrition and well-being: Accessible and enjoyable meals ensure that individuals with dysphagia receive the necessary nutrition for their overall health and well-being. By modifying textures and incorporating a variety of flavors, individuals can maintain a balanced diet and enjoy their meals.
- Quality of life: Dysphagia can significantly impact a person's quality of life, making mealtime a challenging experience. Accessible and enjoyable meals help individuals with dysphagia regain a sense of normalcy, socialize with others, and derive pleasure from eating.
- Inclusion and dignity: Everyone deserves to enjoy meals that align with their dietary needs and preferences. By providing accessible options for individuals with dysphagia, we foster inclusivity and ensure they can participate fully in social

gatherings and family meals.

- Caregiver support: Accessible and enjoyable meals alleviate the burden on caregivers, who play a crucial role in supporting individuals with dysphagia. By providing resources and recipes that simplify meal preparation, we empower caregivers to provide nutritious and satisfying meals with ease.
- Culinary creativity: Creating dysphagia-friendly meals challenges us to think creatively and experiment with different ingredients, textures, and flavors. This not only benefits individuals with dysphagia but also enriches the culinary world by expanding our understanding of food and its potential.

In conclusion, accessible and enjoyable meals for individuals with dysphagia are vital for their nutrition, quality of life, and social well-being. By embracing inclusivity, supporting caregivers, and fostering culinary creativity, we can enhance the dining experiences of individuals with dysphagia and promote a greater sense of joy and fulfillment in their lives.

CHAPTER TWO

Pureed Chicken and Vegetable Soup

Description: This pureed chicken and vegetable soup is a comforting and nourishing meal, perfect for those looking for a smooth and easy-to-digest option. The combination of tender chicken and assorted vegetables creates a flavorful and nutritious blend.

Ingredients:

- 1 boneless, skinless chicken breast
- 2 carrots, peeled and chopped
- 1 celery stalk, chopped
- 1 small onion, diced
- 2 cloves of garlic, minced
- 4 cups low-sodium chicken broth
- 1 bay leaf
- Salt and pepper, to taste

Instructions:

- In a large pot, bring the chicken broth to a boil over medium heat.
- Add the chicken breast, carrots, celery, onion, garlic, and bay leaf to the pot.
- Reduce the heat to low and simmer for about 20 minutes or until the chicken is cooked through and the vegetables are tender.
- Remove the bay leaf from the pot and discard.
- Transfer the cooked chicken breast and vegetables to a blender or food processor. Blend until smooth and creamy.
- Season the pureed soup with salt and pepper to taste.

- Serve hot and enjoy the comforting flavors of this pureed chicken and vegetable soup.

Nutritional Information:

Serving Size: 1 cup

Calories: 150

Total Fat: 4g

Carbohydrates: 10g

Protein: 18g

Soft Scrambled Eggs with Mashed Avocado

Description: Start your day with a satisfying and creamy breakfast of soft scrambled eggs with mashed avocado. This simple yet indulgent dish combines the velvety texture of scrambled eggs with the smoothness of mashed avocado for a delightful morning treat.

Ingredients:

- 4 large eggs
- 1 ripe avocado
- 2 tablespoons milk
- Salt and pepper, to taste
- Fresh chives, for garnish (optional)

Instructions:

- Crack the eggs into a bowl and whisk them together with the milk until well combined.
- Heat a non-stick skillet over medium-low heat.
- Add the egg mixture to the skillet and gently scramble them, stirring continuously with a spatula.
- While the eggs are cooking, peel and pit the

avocado. Mash it with a fork until smooth.

- Season the scrambled eggs with salt and pepper to taste.
- Once the eggs are soft and slightly runny, remove the skillet from heat.
- Transfer the scrambled eggs to a plate and top with a generous dollop of mashed avocado.
- Garnish with fresh chives, if desired.
- Serve immediately and relish the velvety goodness of soft scrambled eggs with mashed avocado.

Nutritional Information:

Serving Size: 1 portion

Calories: 250

Total Fat: 18g

Carbohydrates: 8g

Protein: 14g

Pureed Spinach and Potato Mash

Description: Indulge in a vibrant and creamy pureed spinach and potato mash that will captivate your taste buds. This wholesome blend of spinach and potatoes creates a luxurious texture and a burst of flavors, making it an excellent side dish or a light meal on its own.

Ingredients:

- 2 large potatoes, peeled and diced
- 4 cups fresh spinach leaves
- 2 tablespoons butter
- 1/4 cup milk
- Salt and pepper, to taste

- Nutmeg, for garnish (optional)

Instructions:

- Place the diced potatoes in a pot of salted water and bring it to a boil. Cook until the potatoes are tender.
- Meanwhile, blanch the spinach leaves in boiling water for 1-2 minutes. Drain and set aside.
- Once the potatoes are cooked, drain them and return them to the pot.
- Add the blanched spinach leaves, butter, and milk to the pot with the potatoes.
- Using a potato masher or a fork, mash the potatoes and spinach until smooth and well combined.
- Season the puree with salt and pepper to taste.
- If desired, sprinkle a pinch of nutmeg over the pureed spinach and potato mash for added flavor.
- Serve hot as a side dish or enjoy it as a light and nourishing meal.

Nutritional Information:

Serving Size: 1/2 cup

Calories: 120

Total Fat: 5g

Carbohydrates: 18g

Protein: 3g

Creamy Pureed Butternut Squash Soup

Description: Indulge in the velvety smoothness of creamy pureed butternut squash soup. This comforting soup is bursting with the sweet and nutty flavors of roasted butternut squash, combined with aromatic spices and a touch of cream for a delightful bowl of warmth.

Ingredients:

- 1 medium butternut squash, peeled, seeded, and cubed
- 1 onion, chopped
- 2 cloves of garlic, minced
- 4 cups vegetable broth
- 1/2 teaspoon ground cinnamon
- 1/4 teaspoon ground nutmeg
- 1/2 cup heavy cream
- Salt and pepper, to taste
- Fresh parsley, for garnish (optional)

Instructions:

- Preheat the oven to 400°F (200°C).
- Place the cubed butternut squash on a baking sheet and drizzle with olive oil. Season with salt and pepper.
- Roast the squash in the preheated oven for about 30-35 minutes, or until tender and slightly caramelized.
- In a large pot, sauté the chopped onion and minced garlic until translucent and fragrant.
- Add the roasted butternut squash to the pot along with the vegetable broth, ground cinnamon, and ground nutmeg.
- Bring the mixture to a boil, then reduce the heat and simmer for 15 minutes.
- Using an immersion blender or a regular blender, puree the soup until smooth and creamy.
- Stir in the heavy cream and season with salt and pepper to taste.

- Reheat the soup gently, if needed, and garnish with fresh parsley before serving.

Nutritional Information:

Serving Size: 1 cup

Calories: 180

Total Fat: 10g

Carbohydrates: 22g

Protein: 3g

Soft-Textured Tuna Salad with Mashed Avocado

Description: Enjoy a light and refreshing lunch with this soft-textured tuna salad featuring a creamy twist of mashed avocado. The combination of tender tuna, creamy avocado, and zesty flavors creates a satisfying and healthy meal option.

Ingredients:

- 1 can of tuna, drained
- 1 ripe avocado
- 1 tablespoon Greek yogurt
- 1 tablespoon lemon juice
- 1 tablespoon chopped fresh dill
- Salt and pepper, to taste
- Lettuce leaves, for serving
- Sliced cucumber, for garnish (optional)

Instructions:

- In a bowl, combine the drained tuna, mashed avocado, Greek yogurt, lemon juice, and chopped fresh dill.
- Mix well until all the ingredients are evenly

- incorporated.
- Season the tuna salad with salt and pepper to taste.
- To serve, place lettuce leaves on a plate or in a bowl.
- Spoon the soft-textured tuna salad onto the lettuce leaves.
- Garnish with sliced cucumber, if desired.
- Enjoy this light and satisfying salad as a refreshing meal.

Nutritional Information:

Serving Size: 1 portion

Calories: 220

Total Fat: 15g

Carbohydrates: 7g

Protein: 17g

Pureed Broccoli and Cheddar Cheese Soup

Description: Dive into the comforting flavors of pureed broccoli and cheddar cheese soup. This creamy and nutritious soup combines the goodness of tender broccoli florets with the richness of melted cheddar cheese, creating a bowl of warmth that will leave you craving for more.

Ingredients:

- 2 cups broccoli florets
- 1 small onion, chopped
- 2 cloves of garlic, minced
- 4 cups vegetable broth
- 1 cup shredded cheddar cheese
- 1/2 cup heavy cream

- Salt and pepper, to taste
- Croutons, for garnish (optional)

Instructions:

- In a large pot, sauté the chopped onion and minced garlic until fragrant and translucent.
- Add the broccoli florets to the pot along with the vegetable broth.
- Bring the mixture to a boil, then reduce the heat and simmer for about 10-15 minutes, or until the broccoli is tender.
- Using an immersion blender or a regular blender, puree the soup until smooth.
- Return the pureed soup to the pot and place it over low heat.
- Stir in the shredded cheddar cheese and heavy cream until the cheese is melted and the soup is creamy.
- Season with salt and pepper to taste.
- Reheat the soup gently, if needed, and serve hot.
- Garnish with croutons for added texture and crunch, if desired.

Nutritional Information:

Serving Size: 1 cup

Calories: 220

Total Fat: 15g

Carbohydrates: 10g

Protein: 10g

Mashed Sweet Potatoes with Pureed Chicken

Description: Experience the perfect blend of flavors and

textures with mashed sweet potatoes and pureed chicken. This wholesome combination offers the natural sweetness of sweet potatoes paired with tender and savory pureed chicken, creating a hearty and nutritious dish.

Ingredients:

- 2 large sweet potatoes, peeled and cubed
- 1 boneless, skinless chicken breast
- 1/4 cup chicken broth
- 2 tablespoons butter
- 1/4 cup milk
- Salt and pepper, to taste
- Fresh parsley, for garnish (optional)

Instructions:

- Place the cubed sweet potatoes in a pot of salted water and bring it to a boil. Cook until the sweet potatoes are fork-tender.
- In a separate pot, poach the chicken breast by placing it in the pot with chicken broth and enough water to cover it.
- Bring the pot to a gentle simmer and cook the chicken until it is fully cooked and tender.
- Drain the cooked sweet potatoes and return them to the pot.
- Using a potato masher or a fork, mash the sweet potatoes until smooth.
- Remove the cooked chicken breast from the poaching liquid and transfer it to a blender or food processor. Blend until the chicken is pureed.
- Add the pureed chicken, butter, and milk to the pot with the mashed sweet potatoes.
- Stir well to combine all the ingredients and create a creamy consistency.

- Season with salt and pepper to taste.
- Reheat the mashed sweet potatoes with pureed chicken, if needed, and garnish with fresh parsley before serving.

Nutritional Information:

Serving Size: 1/2 cup

Calories: 180

Total Fat: 8g

Carbohydrates: 18g

Protein: 10g

Pureed Carrot and Ginger Soup

Description: Savor the delightful combination of sweetness from carrots and a hint of warmth from ginger in this pureed carrot and ginger soup. This velvety smooth soup is packed with vitamins and flavors that will invigorate your taste buds and leave you feeling nourished.

Ingredients:

- 4 large carrots, peeled and chopped
- 1 small onion, diced
- 2 cloves of garlic, minced
- 1 tablespoon fresh ginger, grated
- 4 cups vegetable broth
- 1/2 cup coconut milk
- 1 tablespoon olive oil
- Salt and pepper, to taste
- Fresh cilantro, for garnish (optional)

Instructions:

- Heat olive oil in a large pot over medium heat.

- Add the diced onion, minced garlic, and grated ginger to the pot. Sauté until fragrant and the onion is translucent.
- Add the chopped carrots to the pot and sauté for a few minutes to enhance their flavor.
- Pour in the vegetable broth and bring the mixture to a boil. Reduce the heat and simmer for about 15-20 minutes or until the carrots are tender.
- Using an immersion blender or a regular blender, puree the soup until smooth.
- Return the pureed soup to the pot and place it over low heat.
- Stir in the coconut milk and season with salt and pepper to taste.
- Reheat the soup gently, if needed.
- Serve hot and garnish with fresh cilantro for added freshness and color.

Nutritional Information:

Serving Size: 1 cup

Calories: 120

Total Fat: 7g

Carbohydrates: 14g

Protein: 2g

Soft-Textured Meatloaf with Mashed Cauliflower

Description: Indulge in a comforting and satisfying meal of soft-textured meatloaf served alongside creamy mashed cauliflower. This dish brings together the flavors of savory meatloaf and velvety cauliflower for a delightful combination that will make your taste buds dance.

Ingredients:

- 1 pound ground beef
- 1/2 cup breadcrumbs
- 1 small onion, finely chopped
- 2 cloves of garlic, minced
- 1/4 cup milk
- 1 egg, beaten
- 2 tablespoons Worcestershire sauce
- Salt and pepper, to taste
- 1 medium head of cauliflower, cut into florets
- 2 tablespoons butter
- 1/4 cup heavy cream
- Fresh parsley, for garnish (optional)

Instructions:

- Preheat the oven to 375°F (190°C).
- In a large mixing bowl, combine the ground beef, breadcrumbs, chopped onion, minced garlic, milk, beaten egg, Worcestershire sauce, salt, and pepper. Mix well until all the ingredients are evenly incorporated.
- Transfer the meat mixture to a greased loaf pan and press it down evenly.
- Bake the meatloaf in the preheated oven for about 45-50 minutes or until cooked through.
- While the meatloaf is baking, place the cauliflower florets in a pot of salted water. Bring it to a boil and cook until the cauliflower is fork-tender.
- Drain the cooked cauliflower and transfer it to a food processor or blender.
- Add the butter and heavy cream to the cauliflower and blend until smooth and creamy.

- Season the mashed cauliflower with salt and pepper to taste.
- Once the meatloaf is cooked, remove it from the oven and let it rest for a few minutes before slicing.
- Serve the soft-textured meatloaf slices with a side of mashed cauliflower.
- Garnish with fresh parsley, if desired.

Nutritional Information:

Serving Size: 1 slice of meatloaf with 1/2 cup mashed cauliflower

Calories: 350

Total Fat: 24g

Carbohydrates: 12g

Protein: 20g

Creamy Pureed Mushroom Soup

Description: Delight in the earthy and rich flavors of creamy pureed mushroom soup. This velvety smooth soup combines a variety of mushrooms with aromatic herbs and a touch of cream, resulting in a luxurious bowl of comfort that will warm you from the inside out.

Ingredients:

- 1 pound mixed mushrooms (such as cremini, shiitake, and oyster), sliced
- 1 small onion, chopped
- 2 cloves of garlic, minced
- 4 cups vegetable broth
- 1/2 cup heavy cream
- 2 tablespoons butter

- 1 tablespoon chopped fresh thyme
- Salt and pepper, to taste
- Fresh chives, for garnish (optional)

Instructions:

- In a large pot, melt the butter over medium heat.
- Add the chopped onion and minced garlic to the pot. Sauté until fragrant and the onion is translucent.
- Add the sliced mushrooms and chopped fresh thyme to the pot. Cook until the mushrooms have softened and released their juices.
- Pour in the vegetable broth and bring the mixture to a boil. Reduce the heat and simmer for about 15-20 minutes to allow the flavors to meld together.
- Using an immersion blender or a regular blender, puree the soup until smooth and creamy.
- Return the pureed soup to the pot and place it over low heat.
- Stir in the heavy cream and season with salt and pepper to taste.
- Reheat the soup gently, if needed.
- Serve hot and garnish with fresh chives for added freshness and visual appeal.

Nutritional Information:

Serving Size: 1 cup

Calories: 200

Total Fat: 15g

Carbohydrates: 10g

Protein: 5g

Pureed Turkey and Vegetable Casserole

Description: Enjoy a comforting and nourishing casserole made with pureed turkey and a medley of flavorful vegetables. This wholesome dish brings together tender turkey, vibrant vegetables, and a creamy sauce, creating a satisfying meal that will warm both your heart and your stomach.

Ingredients:

- 2 cups cooked turkey, shredded
- 1 cup mixed vegetables (such as carrots, peas, and corn), cooked
- 1 small onion, chopped
- 2 cloves of garlic, minced
- 2 tablespoons butter
- 2 tablespoons all-purpose flour
- 1 cup chicken broth
- 1/2 cup milk
- Salt and pepper, to taste
- Grated cheese, for topping (optional)

Instructions:

- Preheat the oven to 375°F (190°C).
- In a skillet, melt the butter over medium heat.
- Add the chopped onion and minced garlic to the skillet. Sauté until fragrant and the onion is translucent.
- Sprinkle the flour over the onions and garlic. Stir well to combine and cook for a minute to create a roux.
- Slowly pour in the chicken broth and milk, whisking constantly to avoid lumps.
- Cook the sauce until it thickens and becomes

smooth.

- Add the shredded turkey and cooked mixed vegetables to the skillet. Stir well to coat everything with the sauce.
- Season with salt and pepper to taste.
- Transfer the turkey and vegetable mixture to a casserole dish and spread it evenly.
- If desired, sprinkle grated cheese on top for a cheesy crust.
- Bake the casserole in the preheated oven for about 20-25 minutes or until the top is golden and bubbly.
- Serve hot and enjoy the comforting flavors of pureed turkey and vegetables.

Nutritional Information:

Serving Size: 1 cup

Calories: 250

Total Fat: 12g

Carbohydrates: 12g

Protein: 20g

Soft-Textured Salmon Patty with Mashed Peas

Description: Indulge in a delicious and nutritious soft-textured salmon patty served with creamy mashed peas. This delightful combination brings together the delicate flavors of salmon and the vibrant sweetness of peas for a satisfying meal that is both comforting and packed with nutrients.

Ingredients:

- 1 pound fresh salmon fillets, skin removed

- 1/4 cup breadcrumbs
- 1 small onion, finely chopped
- 2 cloves of garlic, minced
- 1/4 cup chopped fresh dill
- 1 egg, beaten
- Salt and pepper, to taste
- 2 cups frozen peas
- 2 tablespoons butter
- 1/4 cup milk
- Fresh lemon wedges, for serving (optional)

Instructions:

- Preheat the oven to 375°F (190°C).
- In a food processor, pulse the salmon fillets until they are finely chopped.
- Transfer the chopped salmon to a mixing bowl and add the breadcrumbs, chopped onion, minced garlic, chopped fresh dill, beaten egg, salt, and pepper. Mix well to combine all the ingredients.
- Shape the salmon mixture into patties of desired size.
- Place the salmon patties on a greased baking sheet and bake in the preheated oven for about 15-20 minutes or until cooked through.
- While the salmon patties are baking, cook the frozen peas according to the package instructions.
- Drain the cooked peas and transfer them to a pot.
- Add the butter and milk to the pot with the peas.
- Using a potato masher or a fork, mash the peas until they reach a smooth and creamy consistency.
- Season the mashed peas with salt and pepper to taste.

- Serve the soft-textured salmon patties with a generous dollop of mashed peas.
- Squeeze fresh lemon juice over the salmon patties, if desired, for a burst of citrus flavor.

Nutritional Information:

Serving Size: 1 salmon patty with 1/2 cup mashed peas

Calories: 280

Total Fat: 15g

Carbohydrates: 15g

Protein: 20g

Pureed Cauliflower and Cheese Soup

Description: Experience the creamy and satisfying flavors of pureed cauliflower and cheese soup. This velvety smooth soup combines the subtle taste of cauliflower with the richness of cheese, resulting in a comforting bowl of goodness that will warm your soul.

Ingredients:

- 1 head cauliflower, cut into florets
- 1 small onion, chopped
- 2 cloves of garlic, minced
- 4 cups vegetable broth
- 1 cup shredded cheddar cheese
- 1/2 cup heavy cream
- 2 tablespoons butter
- Salt and pepper, to taste
- Chopped fresh chives, for garnish (optional)

Instructions:

- In a large pot, melt the butter over medium heat.

- Add the chopped onion and minced garlic to the pot. Sauté until fragrant and the onion is translucent.
- Add the cauliflower florets to the pot and sauté for a few minutes to enhance their flavor.
- Pour in the vegetable broth and bring the mixture to a boil. Reduce the heat and simmer for about 15-20 minutes or until the cauliflower is tender.
- Using an immersion blender or a regular blender, puree the soup until smooth and creamy.
- Return the pureed soup to the pot and place it over low heat.
- Stir in the shredded cheddar cheese and heavy cream until the cheese is melted and the soup is creamy.
- Season with salt and pepper to taste.
- Reheat the soup gently, if needed.
- Serve hot and garnish with chopped fresh chives for added flavor and visual appeal.

Nutritional Information:

Serving Size: 1 cup

Calories: 250

Total Fat: 20g

Carbohydrates: 10g

Protein: 10g

Mashed Lentils with Pureed Spinach

Description: Enjoy a nutritious and flavorful dish of mashed lentils with a vibrant pureed spinach twist. This combination of protein-rich lentils and nutrient-packed spinach creates a satisfying and wholesome meal that will leave you feeling nourished and energized.

Ingredients:

- 1 cup dried lentils
- 2 cups vegetable broth
- 1 small onion, chopped
- 2 cloves of garlic, minced
- 2 cups fresh spinach leaves
- 2 tablespoons olive oil
- Salt and pepper, to taste
- Fresh parsley, for garnish (optional)

Instructions:

- Rinse the dried lentils under cold ater and drain.
- In a pot, combine the lentils, vegetable broth, chopped onion, and minced garlic. Bring to a boil over high heat.
- Reduce the heat to low, cover the pot, and simmer for about 20-25 minutes or until the lentils are tender.
- While the lentils are cooking, bring a separate pot of water to a boil.
- Add the fresh spinach leaves to the boiling water and blanch for 1-2 minutes.
- Drain the spinach and transfer it to a food processor or blender.
- Add the olive oil, salt, and pepper to the spinach.
- Puree the spinach until smooth and creamy.
- Drain the cooked lentils and return them to the pot.
- Mash the lentils using a potato masher or the back of a spoon until they reach a desired consistency.
- Stir in the pureed spinach and mix well to combine.

- Season with additional salt and pepper, if needed.
- Reheat the mashed lentils with pureed spinach gently, if necessary.
- Serve hot and garnish with fresh parsley, if desired, for added freshness and color.

Nutritional Information:

Serving Size: 1 cup

Calories: 200

Total Fat: 8g

Carbohydrates: 25g

Protein: 10g

Soft-Textured Chicken and Rice Porridge

Description: Indulge in a comforting and easy-to-digest meal of soft-textured chicken and rice porridge. This nourishing dish combines tender chicken, delicate rice, and aromatic herbs, creating a soothing bowl of porridge that will warm you from the inside out.

Ingredients:

- 1 cup cooked chicken breast, shredded
- 1/2 cup white rice
- 4 cups chicken broth
- 1 small onion, chopped
- 2 cloves of garlic, minced
- 1 tablespoon grated ginger
- 1 tablespoon soy sauce
- Salt and pepper, to taste
- Chopped green onions, for garnish (optional)

Instructions:

- In a large pot, combine the cooked chicken breast, white rice, chicken broth, chopped onion, minced garlic, grated ginger, and soy sauce.
- Bring the mixture to a boil over high heat.
- Reduce the heat to low, cover the pot, and simmer for about 30-40 minutes or until the rice is soft and the porridge reaches a desired consistency.
- Stir the porridge occasionally to prevent sticking and ensure even cooking.
- Season the porridge with salt and pepper to taste.
- Reheat the porridge gently, if needed.
- Serve hot and garnish with chopped green onions, if desired, for added flavor and freshness.

Nutritional Information:

Serving Size: 1 cup

Calories: 220

Total Fat: 5g

Carbohydrates: 25g

Protein: 20g

CONCLUSION

In conclusion, the Dysphagia Diet serves as a comprehensive guide and empowering resource for individuals navigating the challenges of dysphagia. Through the exploration of various diet textures, modified food and liquid consistencies, and practical strategies, this book equips both patients and caregivers with the knowledge and tools needed to optimize nutrition and enhance quality of life. By embracing a person-centered approach and emphasizing the importance of interdisciplinary collaboration, we can foster a supportive environment that promotes swallowing success and ensures that individuals with dysphagia can savor every meal with confidence. Together, let us continue to champion the importance of dysphagia management, advocate for accessible dining options, and empower those facing swallowing difficulties to lead fulfilling lives filled with joy, nourishment, and connection.